Post Partum Depression

Knowing More about Postnatal Depression

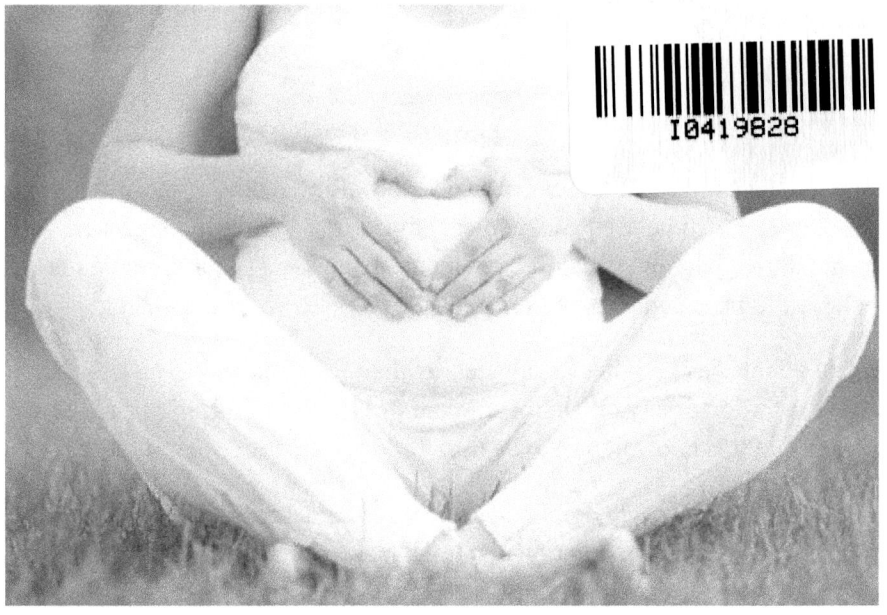

Dueep Jyot Singh

Healthy Learning Series

Mendon Cottage Books

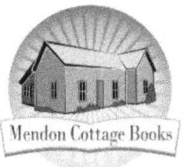

JD-Biz Publishing

Disclaimer

The information is this book is provided for informational purposes only. It is not intended to be used and medical advice or a substitute for proper medical treatment by a qualified health care provider. The information is believed to be accurate as presented based on research by the author.

The contents have not been evaluated by the U.S. Food and Drug Administration or any other Government or Health Organization and the contents in this book are not to be used to treat cure or prevent disease.

The author or publisher is not responsible for the use or safety of any diet, procedure or treatment mentioned in this book. The author or publisher is not responsible for errors or omissions that may exist.

Warning

The Book is for informational purposes only and before taking on any diet, treatment or medical procedure, it is recommended to consult with your primary health care provider.

Download Free Books!

http://MendonCottageBooks.com

Table of Contents

Introduction

It may be an emotional or well-known sentimental cliché that a mother is not really a mother until she has held her baby in her arms, for the first time. Since ancient times, this is the statement which has been followed in societies that a woman can never be fulfilled until she has become a wife and a mother. In fact, nature has programmed a woman to be the mother of future generations, and that is why there is always a feeling that only when she holds her bundle of joy in her arms when she really understand what it really means to be a woman and a mother.

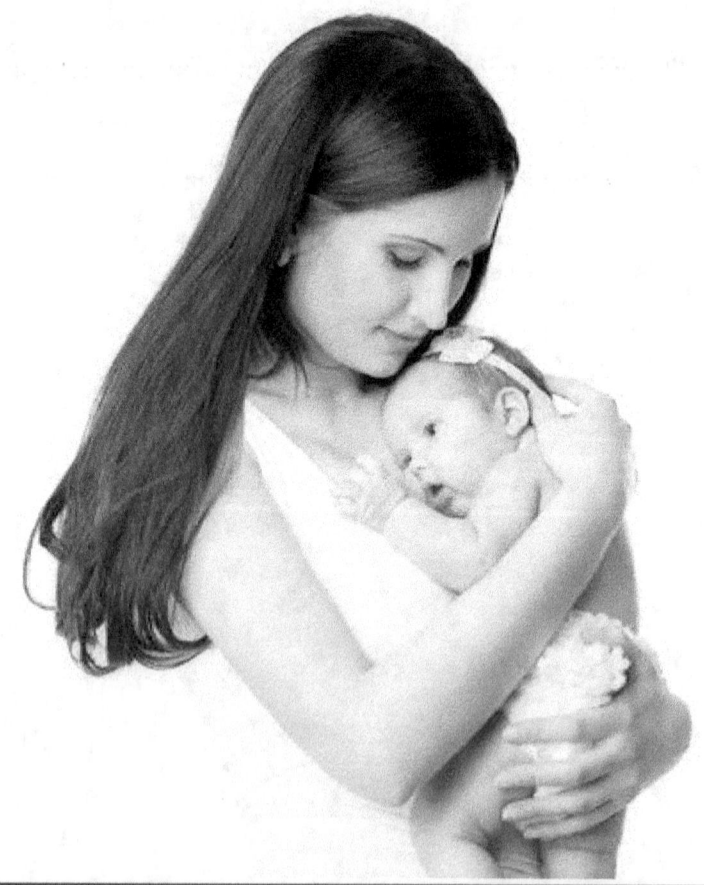

Nevertheless, putting emotion aside, pregnancy and childbirth are going to result in a complex mix of hormonal, physical, emotional, spiritual, and behavioral changes taking place in a woman.

This whole package is going to affect her in various ways at different times. In fact, a woman may recognize the fact that she is expecting, when she finds herself with mood swings in the initial stages of pregnancy. During the pregnancy, she is going to feel excited, full of energy, and deliriously happy. At other times she is going to feel headaches, flustered, and feel tired and overwhelmed.

In the East, since ancient times, women know all about these particular hormonal changes which are going to affect an expectant mother. That is why traditionally an expectant mother was always kept in seclusion with old wise women to take care of her. She was given the task of reading holy books so that her mind could keep calm, peaceful and tranquil. The belief was that in this manner, her child would also be a spiritually rich and enlightened soul.

Naturally, after she has gone through the rigors of labor and has successfully given birth to a child, a woman feels that she has done something marvelous. She has achieved something great, and that is the reason why she cannot stop smiling. Holding her child for the first time in her arms means that now she is ready to take on the responsibility of a brand-new soul who has entered her life and who belongs to her completely.

Later on, the world is going to intrude in her magic world of mother and child and brings with it worry as well as the responsibilities which have now fallen on her shoulders. However, when she knows that she has her family, her partner or her husband who is there to welcome the newborn gift to the world, she is going to feel relieved and less tense and stressed.

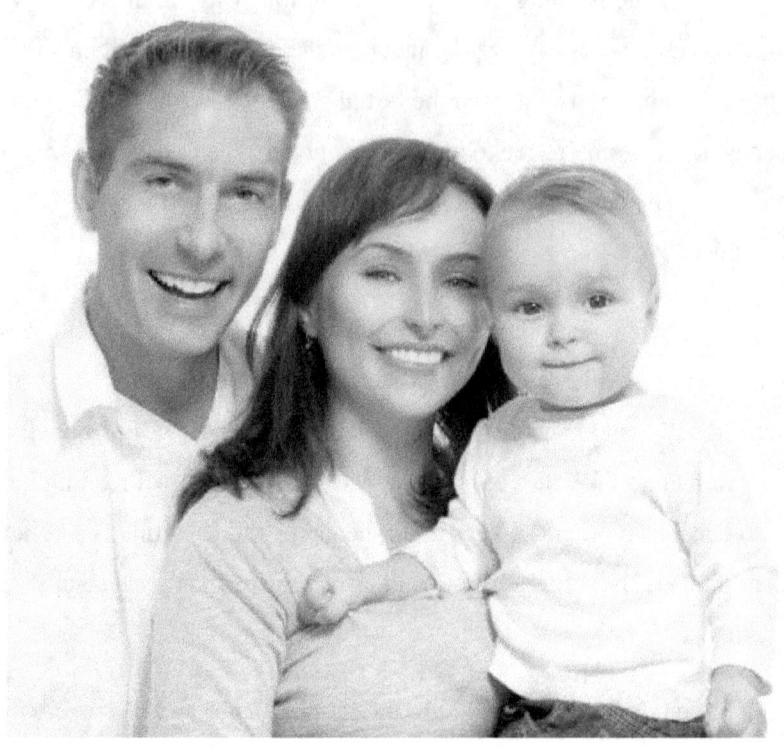

However, a number of women suffer from an ailment known as acute postpartum depression. [PPD.] because of the worry of the responsibility of a newborn child. This makes 90% of the mothers depressed and fearful. But as they begin to cope with baby care, this depression is going to disappear.

Yet for about a quarter of the new mothers, the depression is going to persist for some weeks. They need help in both caring for their babies and in coming to terms with their feelings. It is only with the help and support of their families, that they can manage to come out of this depression.

Acute postpartum depression in a mother is going to result in the baby being badly neglected or even ill treated.

So what is this condition that makes women feel emotionally untouched by their own babies as they drown in a sea of black depression?

Symptoms

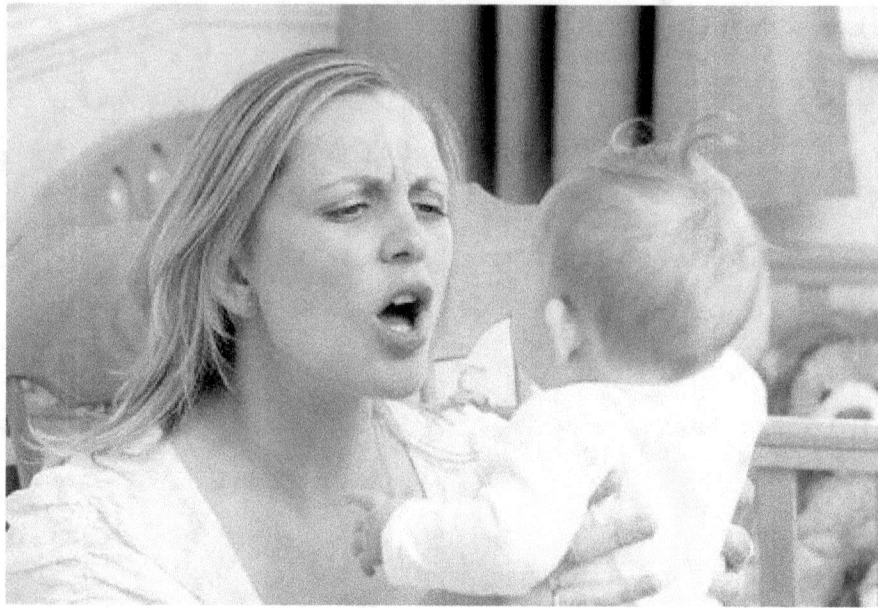

It is important to know that women suffering from postpartum depression should realize that it is an illness like any other ailment of the body. They are not responsible for that condition anyway so they should not feel guilty about their emotions and actions.

A woman suffering from PPD is going to suffer from loss of appetite. She may also become insomniac are perhaps she may start sleeping more than usual. She will lose interest in life, feel depressed and with lower energy levels.

She may also find herself lacking any motivation to get up and do some work, and have crying bouts the same way she had when she was expecting her little one.

Apart from this, she is going to find herself with lower levels of self-confidence and an overwhelming sense of despair, hopelessness, guilt, and even disinterest in the baby.

She may also have something that she might hurt her baby along with panic attacks. Apart from that, she is going to feel worried continuously and constantly. She may also show symptoms of acute and sudden weight loss or weight gain. In some rare cases, they may also turn suicidal.

A dear friend of mine was very thrilled when her son was born and so was the family, because a boy had been born and celebrations, congratulations and jubilation continued for about a month or so after that. And then one day she rang me up and told me that she was not feeling too well and wanted to come back home to her parents, leaving her baby with his father and in the care of her mother-in-law.

When a normally sunny natured person starts speaking of acute depression, wanting to get away from her baby, and so on, I had a feeling that she was suffering from postpartum depression. I immediately told my gynecologist cousin sister-in-law to get to Rena, not as a doctor but as a friend.

Her husband had also seen a change in her personality. In fact, he had started feeling worried about letting the mother alone with her baby, but luckily when my SIL H. spoke to him without his wife's knowledge, naturally he invited her home for lunch one fine day.

H. recognized the symptoms of PPD, thanks to having lots of experience in such cases seen in new mothers in the family owned 30 bed hospital.[1]

The symptoms can start at any time after a baby is born. The former victims of PPD, the symptoms begin soon after childbirth, for some others they may start some weeks or even months later. Occasionally they start even before the baby is born.

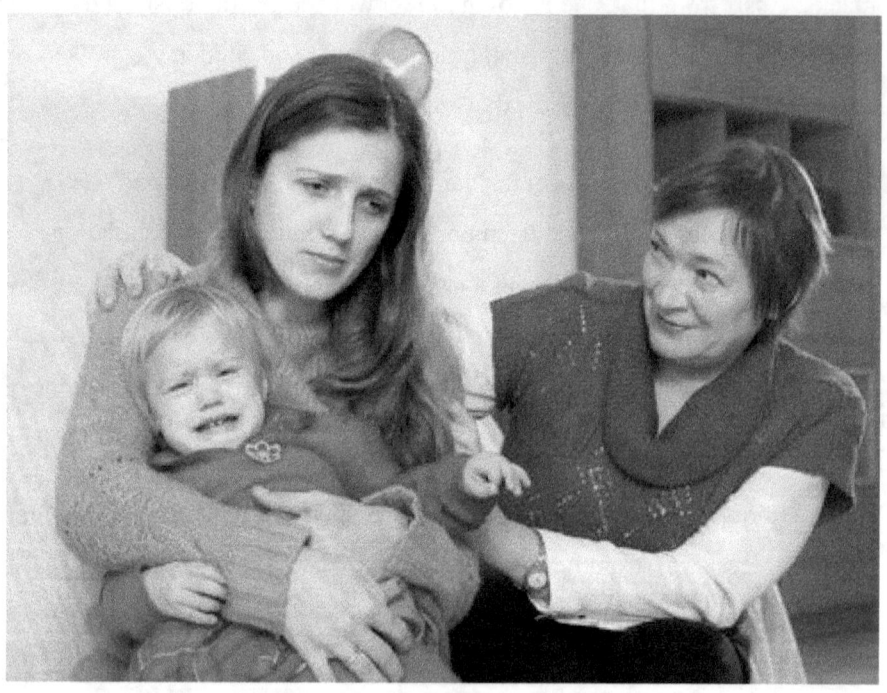

A woman suffering from possible PPD should be given lots of support and care by the people around her.

---

[1] http://www.sharanjithospital.com/

In about .2% of the cases, the mother's negative feelings are so strong that she feels as if the world around her is all black. She also feels that she is drowning in a sea of depression. She feels unable to move and is unwilling to care for her baby because she does not feel any sort of emotional bond with it.

In some cases, she does not want to feed or touch the baby. Rena was in this particular stage, when she did not want anything to do with her baby even feeding it. Unfortunately she had married into a traditional and conservative family, where it was taken for granted that the mother would nurse her child herself. So her mother-in-law was righteously indignant that she had a daughter-in-law who was so unnatural and supposedly "modern."

The mother-in-law did not know anything about PPD. Many women do not. They might quite be capable of calling a depressed mother mad, because she does not want to go near her newborn baby or nurse it.

The name says it all – this depression often occurs after birth and that is why it is either called postpartum or Peripartum depression. In nonmedical terms, this is known as postnatal depression.

Very occasionally usually in very severe cases, the physical and emotional symptoms of acute depression can manifest themselves even before the delivery.

PPD may appear within a few days of giving birth, or may manifest itself more slowly. It may reach the acute stage months after the woman has given birth. It may last from a few weeks to more than a year.

According to H, this depression before delivery can happen when expectant mothers are not really certain about what they are going to face during labor.

They have not been given proper advice by the people around them. Their doctors have also not given them mental and emotional support.

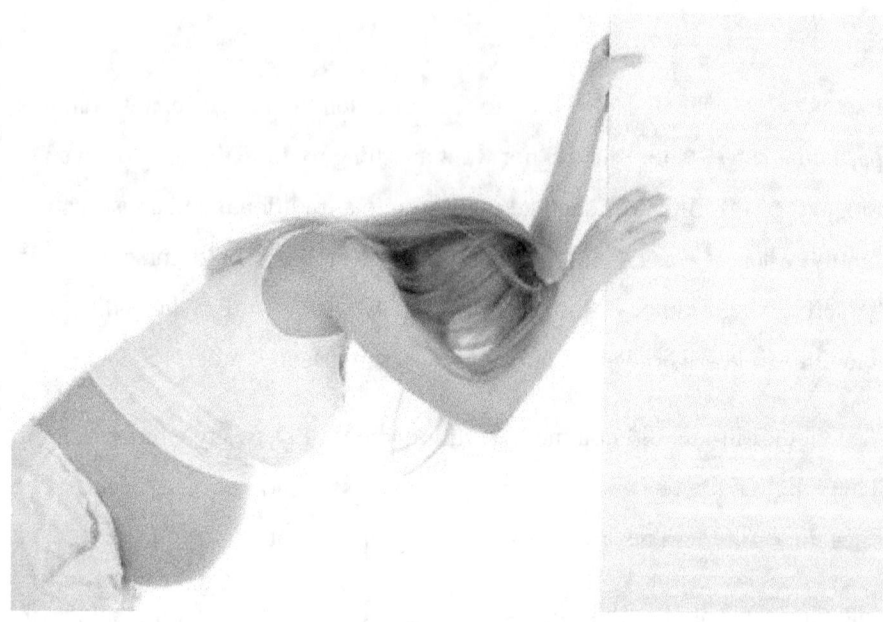

So in such cases, especially when these are first-time mothers, they begin to think of the whole process of childbirth to be something scary, terrifying and horrendous. This is a psychological fear, which manifests itself in depression because fear can grow out of all proportions and have a debilitating effect upon the mind of a young mother.

And if she does not have anybody to allay her fears, give her proper advice, support her, and talk to her in a sensible and mature manner, she is going to spend her time imagining things blown out of all proportion. And this is going to cause even more depression.

In fact, she is going to start blaming her little baby for causing such emotional and mental turmoil in her. She may thus start hating it.

After that she is going to feel guilty because she finds herself having such unnatural feelings towards her child, which according to her, being a mother she should love and so she sinks even more into depression.

A mild version is often called "Having the Baby Blues". The new mother has mood swings. She goes from feeling on top of the world, and then suddenly you might find her weeping. She often feels depressed. She is unable to concentrate on anything she loses her appetite and is unable to sleep soundly.

These symptoms normally start a few days after delivery and are going to last about a week.

Many of us women have gone through this without thinking that this is a symptom of some disorder. We just think that we are overwhelmed by the responsibility that has suddenly been thrust upon us.

In fact, having the blues has been considered such a normal part of early motherhood and the negative feelings that it entails usually go away within a fortnight of delivery.

All this is due to the hormonal changes taking place in the body and the body adapting itself to its new "trial to come."

On the other hand, women suffering from real PPD have more symptoms. The symptoms may also last longer for them. The mild sensation of feeling low and being blue turns into actual depression.

But few people recognize and understand this depression. The mother suffering from it is told in a very strict and bracing tone that she should stop acting babyish and pampering herself. This is normally spoken in strident tones by an elderly woman of the family. Added to that, she is also informed that she should be grateful that she has such a beautiful baby. Also, she should snap out of her bad mood, and fast.

In other words, she is made to feel that she is being self-indulgent, and selfish and hardly anyone understands that her feelings are out of her control.

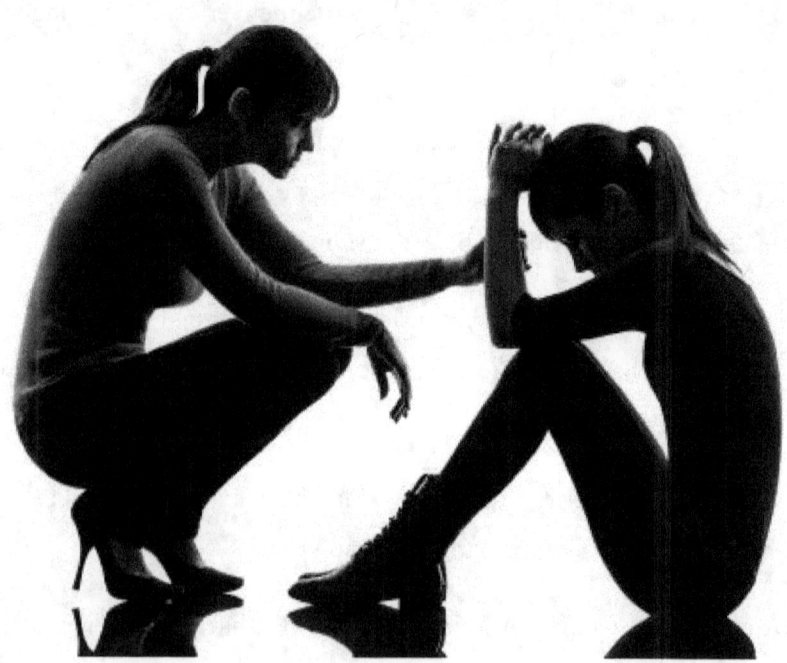

Any sort of depression in anyone is normally seen at first instance as a bid to gain attention and is often dealt with in an inpatient manner.

Believe it or not, I have seen women speaking to their younger relatives in such a bracing tone, and once, even before I knew about PPD, I thought that the new mother was acting melodramatic in order to gain more attention. In fact I had no patience for her, until I got to know more about this particular form of depression.

Causes of PPD

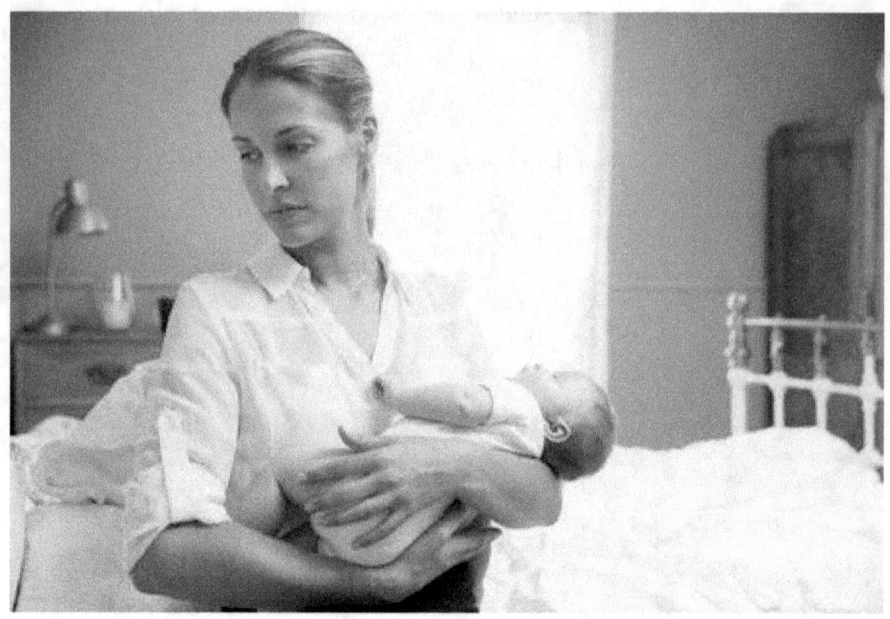

Doctors are still trying to research on the causes of PPD. Why are some mothers capable of raising through pregnancy and childbirth without feeling any sort of depression while others consider this to be a depressing, tiring, and enervating and exhausting phase of their life?

Many researchers have begun to believe that this is possibly due to fluctuating hormonal levels. Again, why hormonal fluctuations take place more in some women and less or not at all in other women is a question that doctors have not been able to answer yet.

But they have noticed that once hormonal levels settle down at normal, pre-pregnancy levels, any sort of depression goes away.

This means that PPD can be treated. This is normally done with antidepressants and hormones.

The hormonal changes that take place during pregnancy and childbirth produce chemical changes in the brain. These cause the basic depression that cause all the other symptoms of PPD. When these absent hormones are supplemented by other hormones, prescribed by your doctor, the body and the brain is going to find them enough in order to keep functioning in a normal and healthy manner.

However, the treatment may not always work well and the real cure is when the body suddenly decides to snap out of it and come back to normal. This happened to my friend Rena, who apart from suffering from PPD was also suffering from a cute case of mother-in-law ness. Her exhortations, views and counsels were quite enough to make Rena. feel even more depressed.

Until one fine day, she woke up in the morning, because she had had a nightmare. Her baby was dead through her negligence. She woke up screaming, because she would not accept that fact, would not believe it, and suddenly her mind snapped out of that depression. She has two sons now, and she has had absolutely no other attacks of PPD. And she is also a loving and caring mother.

I know of another friend, who was suffering from an acute case of PPD. She began to suffer from tremors, chest pain, dizziness and headaches, at the mere thought of holding and nursing her child. She was not able to sleep and the doctor prescribed sleeping pills for her. She took them, but they hardly helped her case.

A week passed and then another and her condition began to deteriorate. She began to get upset by noises, and even the normal sounds of conversation and vehicles passing on the roads outside disturbed her.

She shut the door to her room, drew the curtains, and asked that no one come in. She stopped eating because she did not feel hungry at all.

Her mother was there as well as her mother-in-law and sister-in-law to help take care of the baby. They encouraged her in the initial stages to take rest and get her health back, but as her depression worsened, the ladies of the family began to lose patience with her.

In fact, she reached the stage when she did not want to hold her baby, feed him, rocking to sleep or have anything to do with him. If she was forced to have anything to do with the baby, – especially at times when her mother, mother-in-law or sister-in-law were busy in other jobs – she felt like throwing him down. Sadly enough, this is an acute case, where the mother starts to get frightened that she may harm her baby one day.

That is when she is going to begin to dread the times when her child was brought to her to be fed. She may also, if she is sensible begin to find her own behavior bizarre and unnatural. Her depression is going to worsen and she is going to ask herself if she was abnormal.

If she was not abnormal, why does not she want to feed or hold the child she had awaited so eagerly? She may also think that she is going mad.

Doctor, Can You Please Help Me?

Now for my friend, she went for her routine checkups and told the doctor about her physical problems, the loss of appetite, the headaches, the dizziness, the constant fatigue, and the occasional pain in the chest.

I am sorry to say but the doctor did not take them seriously. She only just made reassuring noises, and told her that she was taking longer than most new mothers to recover from the birth of the baby. She then prescribed some tonics and supplements and told my friend to force herself to eat. She owed it to her baby to be healthy enough to take care of him.

My friend came home from these checkups feeling guilty and desperate.

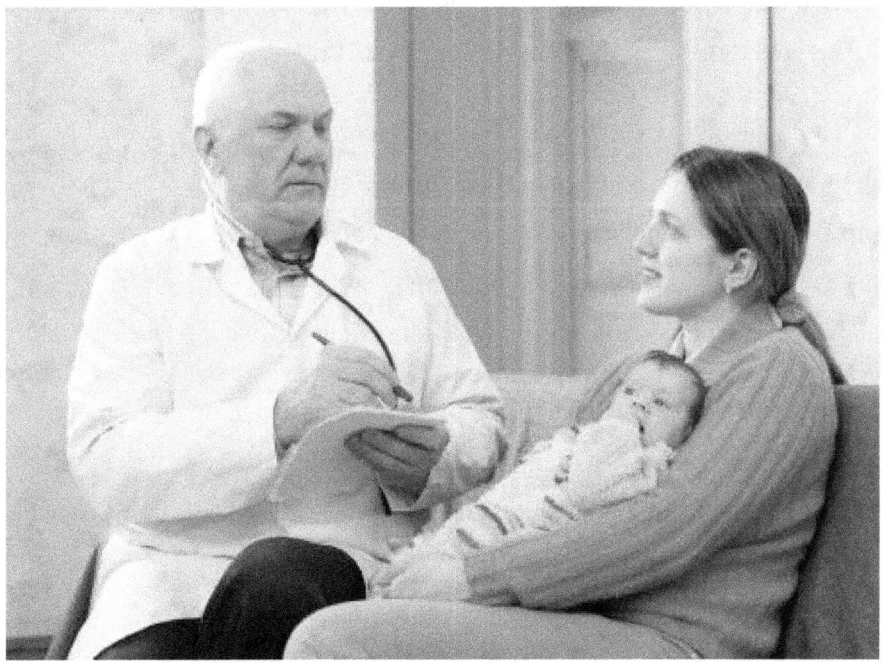

It is possible that the doctor could have diagnoses the symptoms of acute PPD, if my friend had told her about her emotional disturbances. But the answer was that my friend did not want to tell the doctor that she felt ashamed about her negative feelings for her little one. According to her, this proved that she was not a normal woman…

My friend's condition worsened over the next month and her family members began to get worried. They realize that she was not suffering from weakness, but they thought that she was having some sort of nervous breakdown and they did not know why.

Even a change of location, away from the responsibility of the baby did not have any signal effect on her condition. She could not eat or sleep. Her hands trembled. She had attacks of dizziness and severe headaches. Also, she did not want anything to do with her baby which worried her husband even more. Luckily, he noticed her reluctance to hold her baby and one day he suggested that they should consult a Psychiatrist.

She immediately vetoed the idea because according to her, the idea of going to a psychiatrist was something shocking and disgraceful and would only prove that she was not mentally, spiritually and emotionally healthy. Her husband being a sensible person reassured her that talking to a Psychiatrist about her emotional problems was not something of which to be ashamed.

Luckily, the psychiatrist recognized her symptoms and told her all about PPD. He explained to my friend and her family the reasons why she was feeling so depressed. In fact, her mother-in-law, who had accompanied her son and daughter-in-law to the doctor and had half a century's experience with pregnancy and childbirth had never heard of anything like it!

According to her, yes, some women became panicky, were not able to sleep and were down in the dumps and worried for some time, but they snapped out of it in a few weeks. So, it naturally came as a shock that this was some sort of disorder and ailment, and her daughter-in-law was suffering from a severe form of PPD.

Just this little bit of knowledge and information was enough to relieve my friend so much that she felt that a burden had been lifted from her shoulders. She was not mad. She was not abnormal. She certainly did not hate her baby and she would best of all definitely get better.

Just imagine the feeling of acute euphoria and happiness felt by a mother, who understand that what she is feeling is a sickness, and not something psychologically, emotionally or mentally wrong with her.

She would not have gone through all this trauma if she and the people around her had been aware of what PPD really was. PPD actually disappeared by itself. There was no such treatment for postpartum depression which was controlled by antidepressants, occasionally hormones, and sleeping pills. These were just to help the mother cope with the symptoms. Until the PPD disappeared, the mother needed to be helped with baby care.

My friend began to take antidepressants, and slowly within a year, she began to see signs of improvement. She felt less tired and began to sleep soundly for a few ours every night. One day she realized that she had slept deeply throughout the night.

This immediately made her feel so happy that her mind had begun shaking off the depression. Her mother-in-law took care of the baby, because she says that until her daughter-in-law snapped out of the depression, she would be better off not being around her little one.

One night the little baby started crying, and woke the mother up. She kept waiting for someone to come in pick the baby up and shush it. But no one came there and the baby continue to cry. She sat up, swung her legs off the bed and walked to the room, where her baby was crying in a fretful tone of voice. She picked him up, and began to shush him. "Shhhh, my baby", she said softly, "Your mama is here to take care of you, do not you cry anymore."

She heard a noise at the door and turned, to see her mother-in-law standing there weeping with joy. Since then, she never looked back. Her improvement was rapid. That is because her mind had slowly begun to accept the fact that it was time it went back to its pre-pregnancy self and state of levelheaded, calm, and tranquil equanimity.

My friend's little one is now 10 years old. And his mom is back to her state of hearty cheerfulness.

When Brooke Shields went public with her own struggles with postpartum depression, her audience was stunned because even in the West, with its scientific development and research into such problems, many women had not heard of it. In fact, many people accuse her of just being a spoiled attention seeker.

However, with the passing of time, more and more people are getting to know all about this disorder. The mother is not an attention seeker. In fact, she is requesting for help and support in order to get past that depression.

My friend was lucky that she had people who stood by her and helped her through her ordeal imagine what would have happened if she had been by herself or if her husband, parents and in-laws had been less supportive, considering her to be a melodramatic, neurotic, and self-indulgent spoiled brat.

Who Can Get PPD? – Risk factors

Though any woman who is expecting or who has had a child recently can possibly suffer from PPD, some are more at risk than others. These include those women who may be undergoing some sort of stress in their marriage. Also, these women may have family members to they are not so close and they have no one with whom they can talk freely.

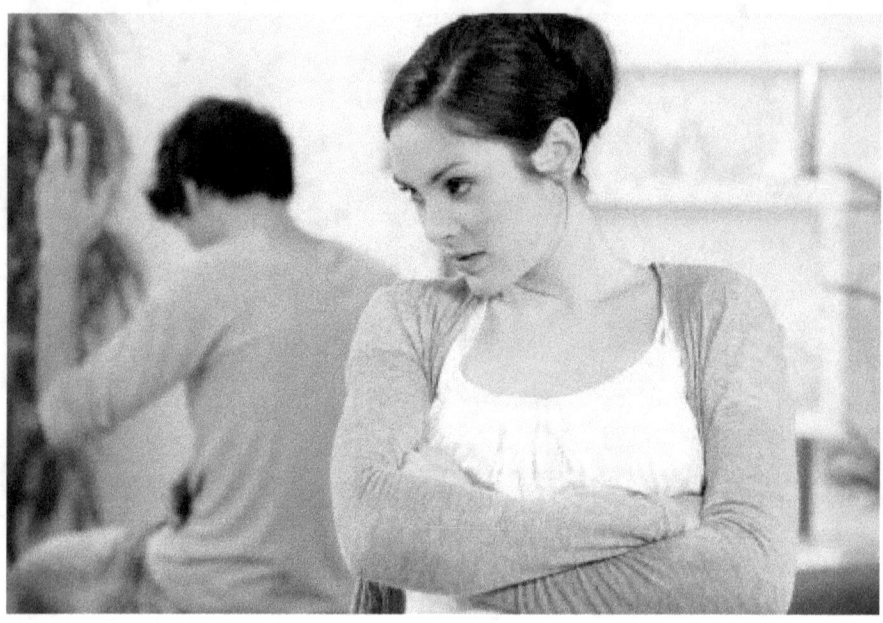

Women who suffer from severe PMS are also at higher risk because they already have hormonal problems. In the same manner, women who have suffered from PPD after the birth of earlier children are who have suffered from depression earlier in any form are also at higher risk.

Stressful events like a divorce, the death of a close relative or a friend, etc. can also increase risk of PPD.

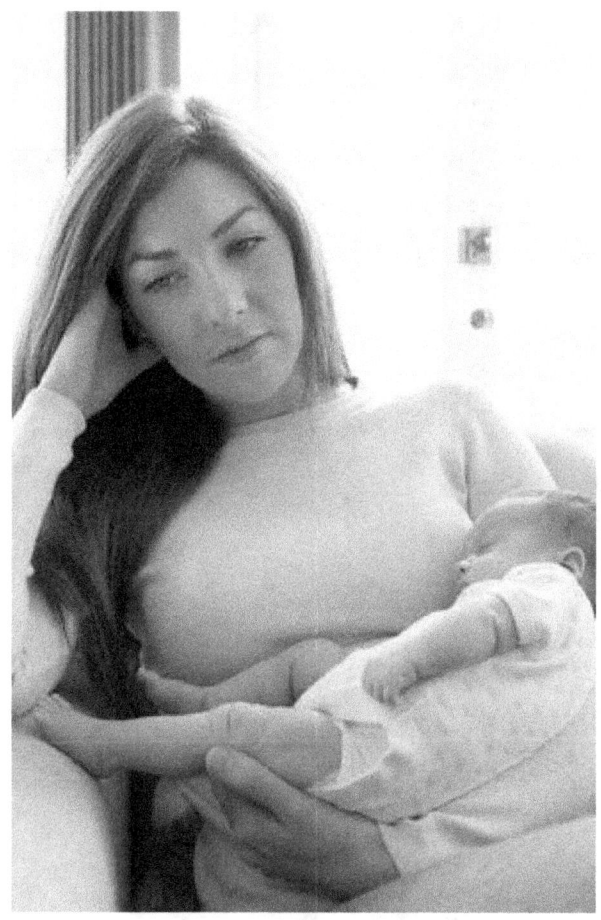

The chances of first-time mothers getting it is more than women who have already gone through the ordeal of childbirth.

Suffering from PPD

If you find yourself suffering from PPD, tell yourself that you are not the first and will not be the last to suffer in this fashion. You do not hate your baby, you are not going mad. So do not keep quiet because you feel guilty.

Talk to someone you trust about your feelings and symptom. If yours is a severe case, you will need to see a doctor or a psychiatrist immediately. Even if yours is not a severe case, you still must not take it too lightly, because any sort of depression is not a healthy condition in which a mother should be in.

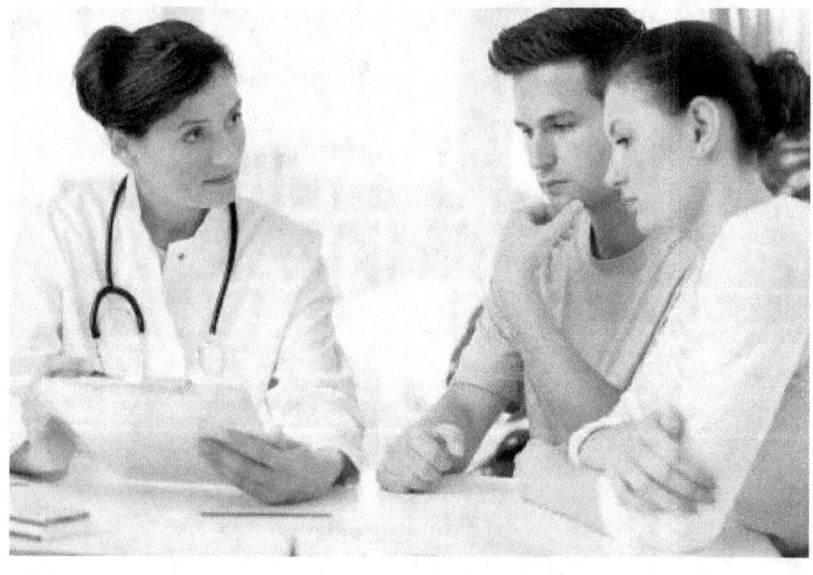

You may possibly like your husband to be with you, when you go and talk to your doctor so that he can understand about PPD and your psychological, mental, and emotional state of mind.

You may also want to explain the situation to your husband and ask him to help you with the baby or with the housework until you regain your energy. You may also want to request are relative to come and help you for a while. Take your mind off your problems by reading, going for walks, exercising, and meditating.

There was a time when women suffering from PPD were considered to be self-indulgent, and lazy, because they were not snapping out of their state of lethargy, mental and physical. You may want to tell yourself this. You are not self-indulgent. However, you do not want to coddle your ailment and allow it to be the focus – be-all and end-all – of your life. So get some other interests, which are going to stop you from brooding over your state of mind.

That means you are going to tell yourself repeatedly that you are going through something that is quite normal for a woman in many cases. You are after all, trying to come to terms with something overpowering and overwhelming. You are now responsible for another human being.

You are a mother and if your body does not cooperate with you, things can become a little too much to cope with for a while. That is why you need to train your mind to accept the fact that your body is strong and your mind is strong.

Duration

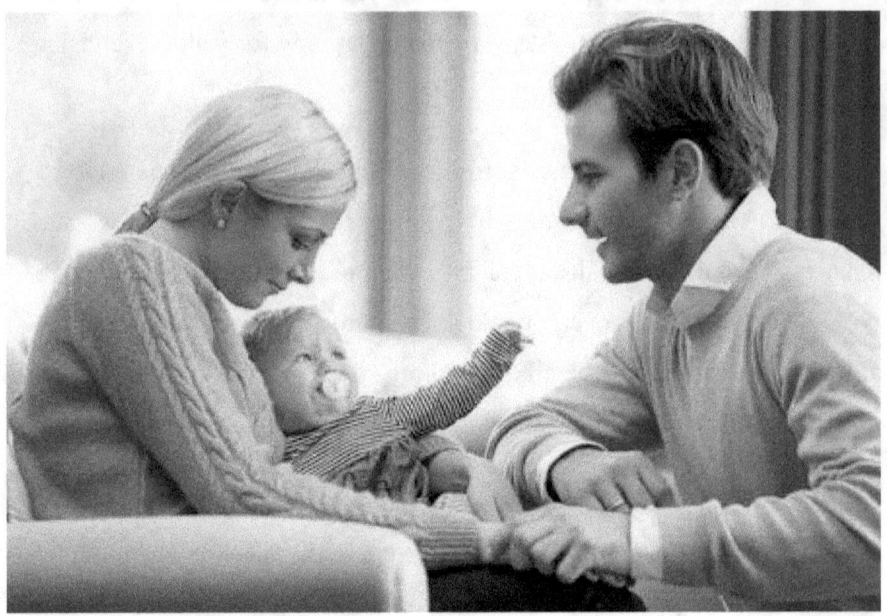

The support of your family members can be enough to help you get out of this state of depression.

PPD can continue from the period of one week or so to some months or even more than a year. This is going to go away as the body comes back to its state of good health, and the hormone levels start coming back to normal slowly and steadily.

PPD can be treated with therapy or medicines. Just talking to a person who has suffered from PPD herself can also help, especially in forums or group sessions. That is because the mother can get reassured that she is not abnormal nor is she suffering from an ailment which is going to linger on throughout her life.

I remember reading one of the historical novels written by Jo Beverley, where Beowulf Malloren who is the Marquess of Rothgar does not intend to get married at all. That is because he has seen his mother strangling her newborn baby when he was five years old. Everybody believed that she was mad, because even though she was suffering from an acute case of PPD, but 300 years ago, nobody knew about it.

They just decided that she had inherited the gene of madness from her side of the family, and when she committed suicide, it was considered to be on par for the course.

Luckily in the 21st century, newborn mothers do not have to face the calumny of being considered mad if they feel depressed or do not want to see their babies. Doctors should be experienced enough to recognize the symptoms, and not treat it casually as something being exaggerated by the patient in order to gain some attention.

If you are nursing your child, you should tell the doctor this, so that she does not prescribe any antidepressants or any other strong medications for you, in case the child is harmed.

Conclusion

This book has given you plenty of information about postpartum depression, and how women suffering from this ailment can manage to snap out of it in a proper manner.

The reason why this ailment has been neglected for so long down the centuries is because of social, conventional and traditional reasons. It has been an instinct of women not to talk about their personal problems or ailments with anybody, especially in the presence of men down the ages.

The idea of repressed Victorian women talking about childbirth in front of menfolk – even their doctors – would be enough to make them swoon. That is the reason why the doctors did not know much about women's ailments, because the women were too shy, too repressed, or to inhibited to talk about them.

Even today, in many parts of the world, women do not talk about women's ailments, in front of men. In fact, they want to pretend that men do not know anything about women's ailment. And the men also being rather shy and brought up in a particular fashion, pretend they do not know about the natural body functions which a woman undergoes during her life, especially during childbirth.

When they are faced with reality, especially with this modern trend of fathers being present in the labor room, it is no wonder that men have also begun to show stress and tension, especially when their wives are expecting.

So, recent research has shown that after becoming fathers, men too have a tendency to suffer from depression. They may also suffer from symptoms similar to those which a woman with PPD suffers from! People reading this may scoff, but it is reality.

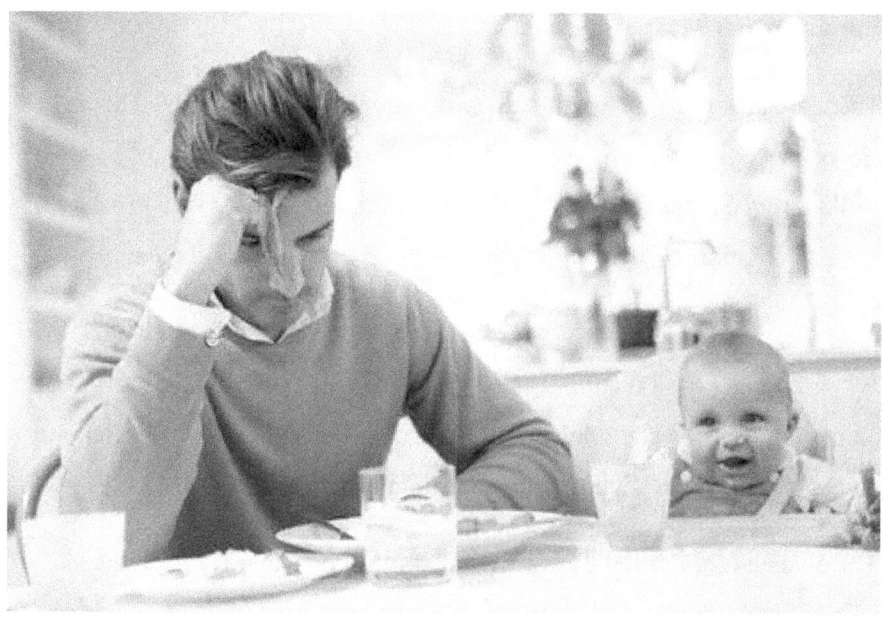

Fathers can also feel depressed with the added responsibilities and stresses of a baby!

This is usually caused by the pressures of increased responsibility, sudden realization of a change in lifestyle, increased expectations, decreased sleep, worry, confusion, tension, and stress related to the realization of what being a father really means.

This normally takes place in responsible men, who have suddenly grown up and woken up to the fact that they are now fathers and now have the responsibility of a baby in their midst.

Many of them are just going to fold up under the burden. And they are going to suffer from the stress. They now understand the upheaval that a baby brings about in a home. Also, they are going to face an increased burden of work and responsibility and tension, if the mother also happens to be suffering from PPD or ill health.

There are absolutely no hormonal and chemical changes involved here. However, these problems are psychological and psychosomatic. It has been well known that the depression and other symptoms bear witness that men are also emotionally and spiritually as well as physically and mentally vulnerable at this particular time.

When I was a hospital administrator in my cousin's hospital, I often saw many of these expectant fathers in an even worse condition physically and mentally, than their wives in the labor room.

The clichéd idea of the father pacing nervously on a corridor, and then calmly handing out cigars when the baby is born is old hat and romantic fiction or filmdom stuff. In reality, he may possibly suffer from phantom labor pains, stress, tension, bad temper, headaches, nausea, dizziness and other symptoms which normally are symptomatic of PPD!

So I would not be surprised that one fine day, a man may be given paternity leave when and after his wife gives birth to a child in order to recuperate from Male PPD!

Live Long and Prosper!

Author Bio

Dueep Jyot Singh is a Management and IT Professional who managed to gather Postgraduate qualifications in Management and English and Degrees in Science, French and Education while pursuing different enjoyable career options like being an hospital administrator, IT,SEO and HRD Database Manager/ trainer, movie , radio and TV scriptwriter, theatre artiste and public speaker, lecturer in French, Marketing and Advertising, ex-Editor of Hearts On Fire (now known as Solstice) Books Missouri USA, advice columnist and cartoonist, publisher and Aviation School trainer, ex-moderator on Medico.in, banker, student councilor ,travelogue writer … among other things!

One fine morning, she decided that she had enough of killing herself by Degrees and went back to her first love -- writing. It's more enjoyable! She already has 48 published academic and 14 fiction- in- different- genre books under her belt.

When she is not designing websites or making Graphic design illustrations for clients , she is browsing through old bookshops hunting for treasures, of which she has an enviable collection – including R.L. Stevenson, O.Henry, Dornford Yates, Maurice Walsh, De Maupassant, Victor Hugo, Sapper, C.N. Williamson, "Bartimeus" and the crown of her collection- Dickens "The Old Curiosity Shop," and "Martin Chuzzlewit" and so on… Just call her "Renaissance Woman") - collecting herbal remedies, acting like Universal Helping Hand/Agony Aunt, or escaping to her dear mountains for a bit of exploring, collecting herbs and plants and trekking.

Check out some of the other JD-Biz Publishing books

Gardening Series on Amazon

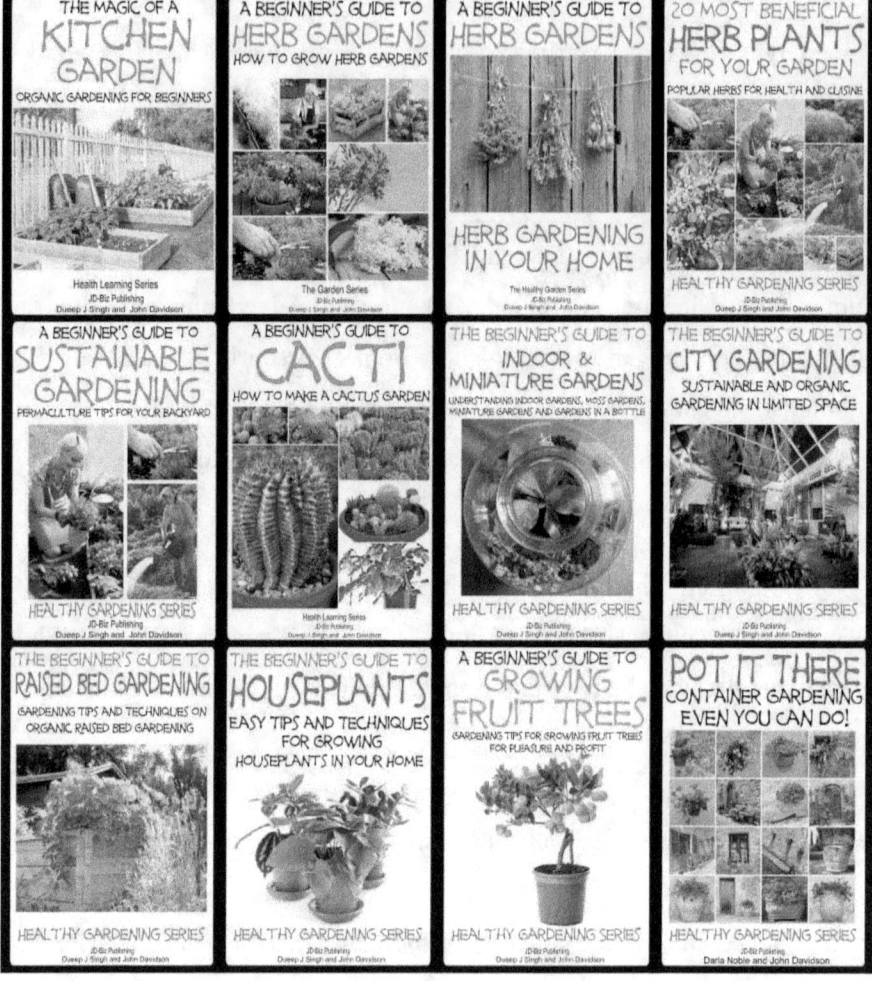

Health Learning Series

THE MAGIC OF **GOOSEBERRIES** FOR HEALTH AND BEAUTY — Natural Remedy Series, JD-Biz Publishing, Dueep J Singh and John Davidson

THE MAGIC OF **YOGURT** FOR COOKING AND BEAUTY — Natural Remedy Series, JD-Biz Publishing

THE MAGIC OF **LEMONS** USING LEMONS FOR HEALTH AND BEAUTY — Natural Remedy Series, JD-Biz Publishing

THE MAGIC OF **CHILLIES** FOR COOKING AND HEALING — Natural Remedy Series, JD-Biz Publishing

THE MAGIC OF **ONIONS** ONIONS IN CUISINE TO CURE AND TO HEAL — Natural Remedy Series, JD-Biz Publishing, Dueep J Singh and John Davidson

THE MAGIC OF **RADISHES** TO CURE AND TO HEAL — Natural Remedy Series, JD-Biz Publishing, Dueep J Singh and John Davidson

THE MAGIC OF **CARROTS** TO CURE AND TO HEAL — Natural Remedy Series, JD-Biz Publishing, Dueep J Singh and John Davidson

THE HEALTH BENEFITS OF **OREGANO** FOR COOKING AND HEALTH — Natural Remedy Series, JD-Biz Publishing, M. Usman and John Davidson

THE MAGIC OF **MARIGOLDS** Marigolds for Health And Beauty — Natural Remedy Series, JD-Biz Publishing, Dueep J Singh and John Davidson

THE HEALTH BENEFITS OF **CINNAMON** — Natural Remedy Series, JD-Biz Publishing, M. Usman and J. Davidson

THE MAGIC OF **COCONUTS** FOR COOKING & HEALTH — Health Learning Series, JD-Biz Publishing, Dueep J Singh and John Davidson

THE MAGIC OF **CLOVES** FOR HEALING AND COOKING — Health Learning Series, JD-Biz Publishing, Dueep J Singh and John Davidson

THE MAGIC OF **ASAFETIDA** FOR COOKING AND HEALING — Health Learning Series, JD-Biz Publishing, Dueep J Singh and John Davidson

THE MAGIC OF **NEEM** MARGOSA TO HEAL — Natural Remedy Series, JD-Biz Publishing, Dueep J Singh and John Davidson

THE MAGIC OF **SALT** TO HEAL AND FOR BEAUTY — Natural Remedy Series, JD-Biz Publishing, Dueep J Singh and John Davidson

THE MAGIC OF **POMEGRANATES** FOR HEALTH AND BEAUTY — Natural Remedy Series, JD-Biz Publishing, Dueep J Singh and John Davidson

THE MAGIC OF **DRY FRUIT AND SPICES** REMEDIES AND RECIPES — Natural Remedy Series, JD-Biz Publishing, Dueep J Singh and John Davidson

THE HEALTH BENEFITS OF **TURMERIC CURCUMIN** FOR COOKING AND HEALTH — Natural Remedy Series, JD-Biz Publishing, M. Usman and J. Davidson

THE MAGIC OF **ALOE VERA** — Natural Remedy Series, JD-Biz Publishing, Dueep J Singh and John Davidson

THE MAGIC OF **VEGETABLES** ANCIENT HEALING REMEDIES AND TIPS — Natural Remedy Series, JD-Biz Publishing, Dueep J Singh and John Davidson

THE HEALTH BENEFITS OF **ROSEMARY** FOR COOKING AND HEALTH — Natural Remedy Series, JD-Biz Publishing, M. Usman and J. Davidson

THE MAGIC OF **PEPPER & PEPPERCORNS** FOR COOKING & HEALING — Natural Remedy Series, JD-Biz Publishing, Dueep J Singh and John Davidson

THE MAGIC OF **MILK, BUTTER AND CHEESE** FOR COOKING & HEALING — Natural Remedy Series, JD-Biz Publishing, Dueep J Singh and John Davidson

THE MAGIC OF **CARDAMOMS** FOR COOKING AND HEALTH — Health Learning Series, JD-Biz Publishing, Dueep J Singh and John Davidson

THE HEALTH BENEFITS OF **BLACK CUMIN** FOR COOKING AND HEALTH — Natural Remedy Series, JD-Biz Publishing, M. Usman and J. Davidson

THE MAGIC OF **BASIL-TULSI** TO HEAL NATURALLY — Health Learning Series, JD-Biz Publishing, Dueep J Singh and John Davidson

THE MAGIC OF **SPICES** FOR HEALTH AND CUISINE — Natural Remedy Series, JD-Biz Publishing, Dueep J Singh and John Davidson

THE MAGIC OF **ROSES** FOR COOKING AND BEAUTY — Natural Remedy Series, JD-Biz Publishing, Dueep J Singh and John Davidson

The Miraculous Healing Powers of **GINGER** — Natural Remedy Series, JD-Biz Publishing, Dueep J Singh and John Davidson — BEST

The Miracle of **HONEY** — Natural Remedy Series, JD-Biz Publishing, Dueep J Singh and John Davidson — BEST

Country Life Books

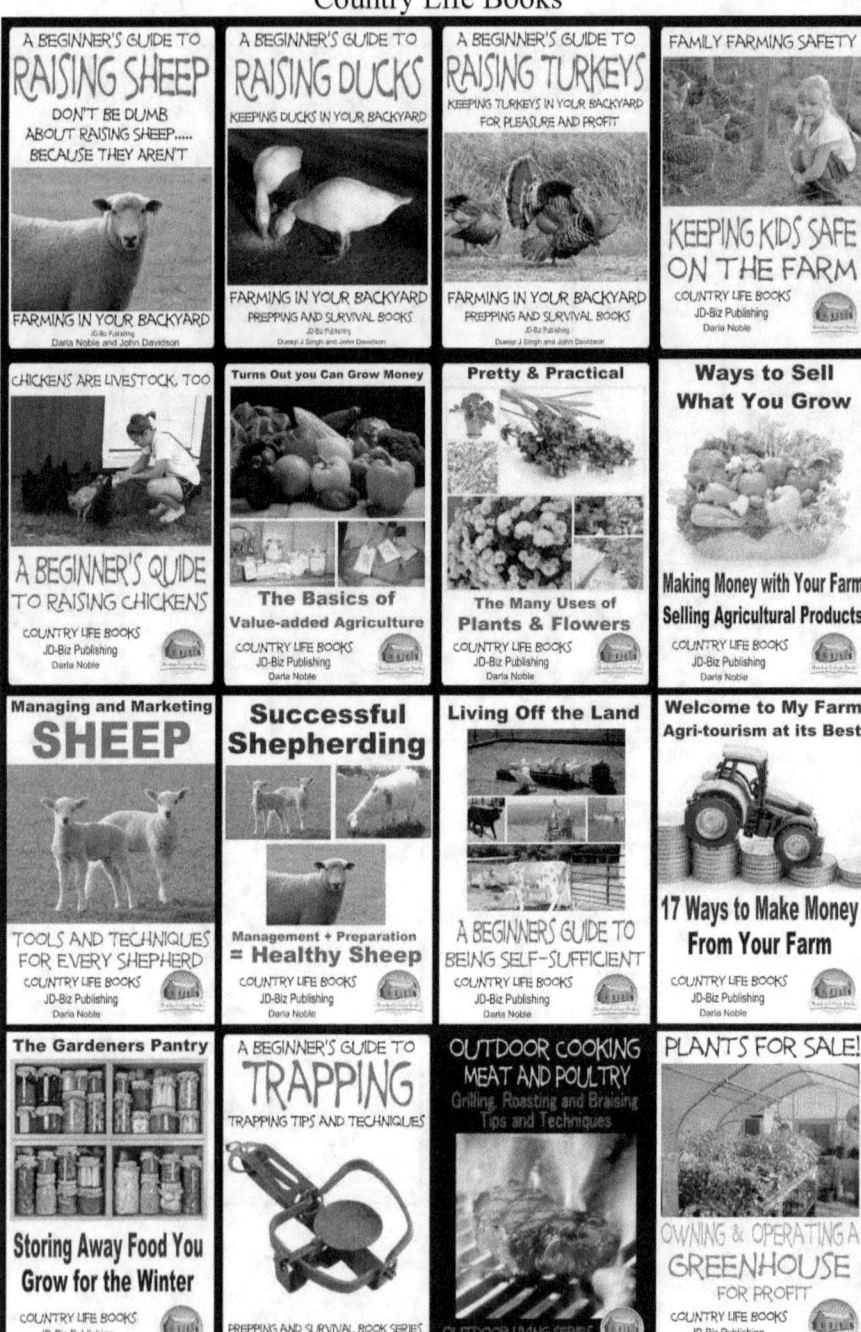

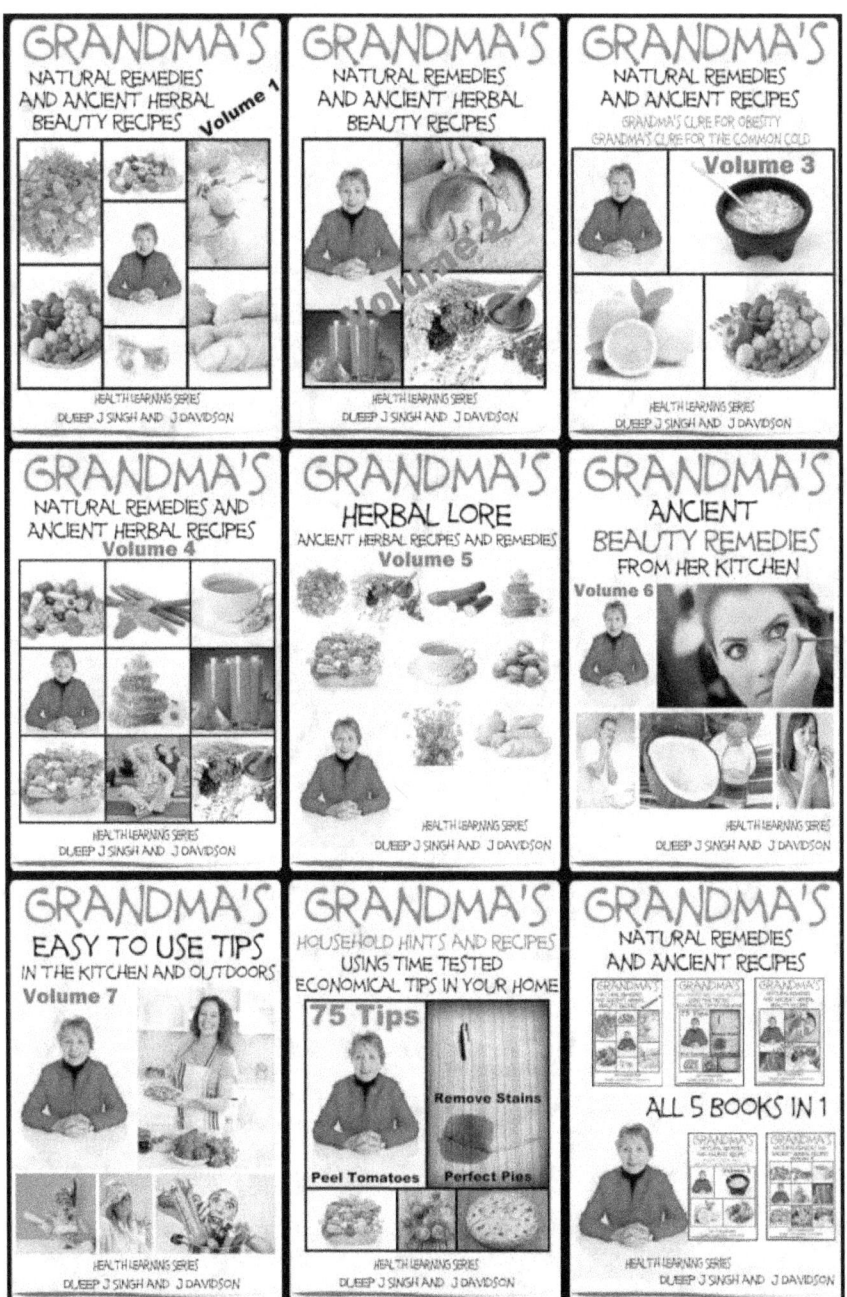

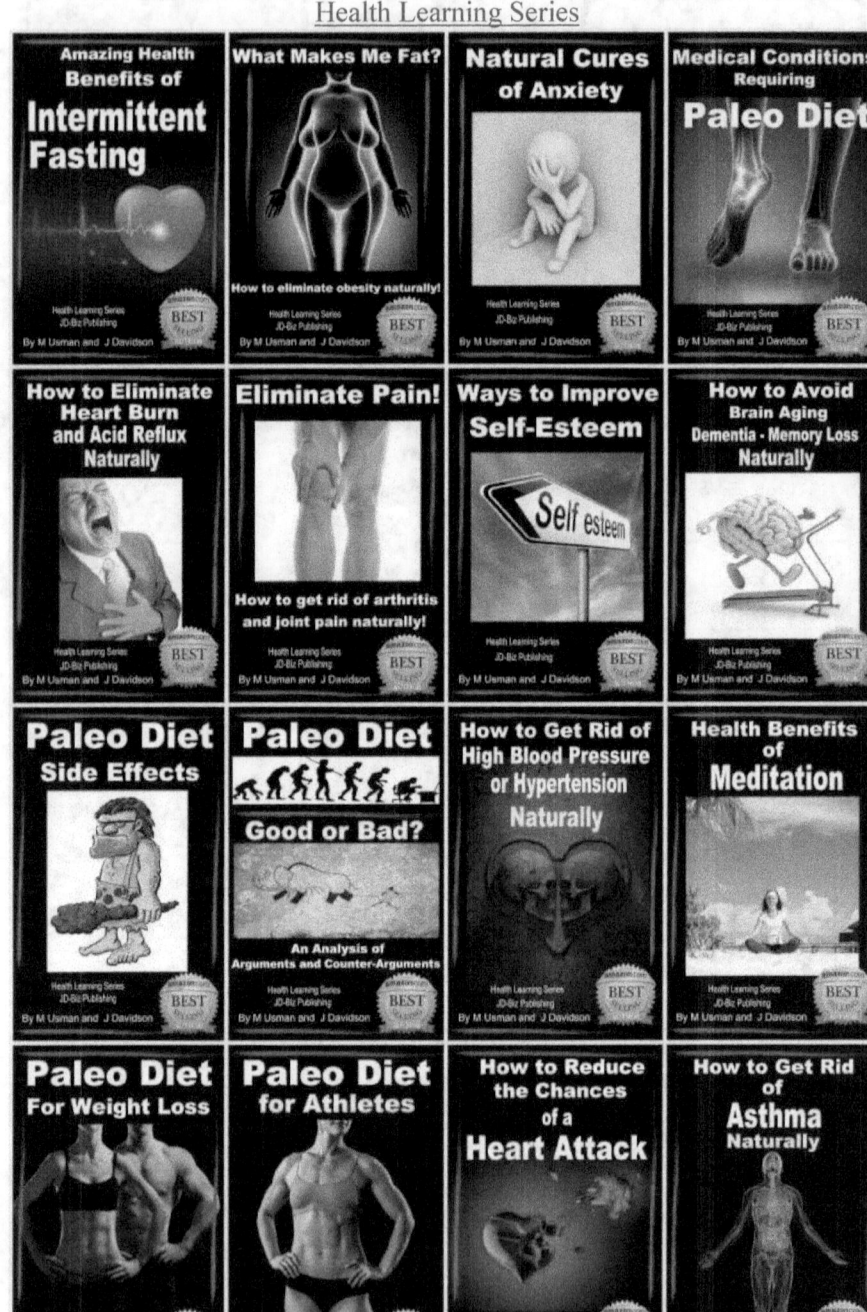

Amazing Animal Book Series

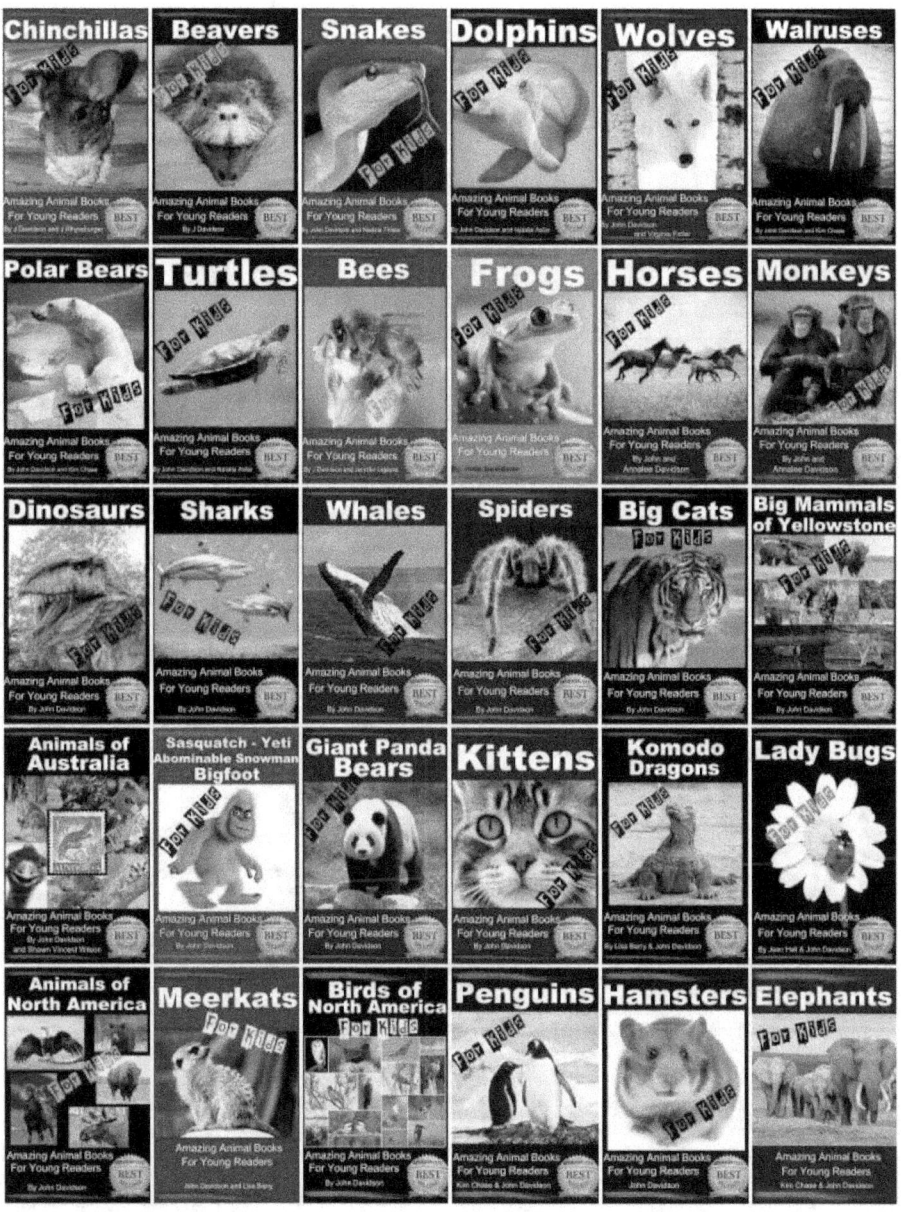

Learn To Draw Series

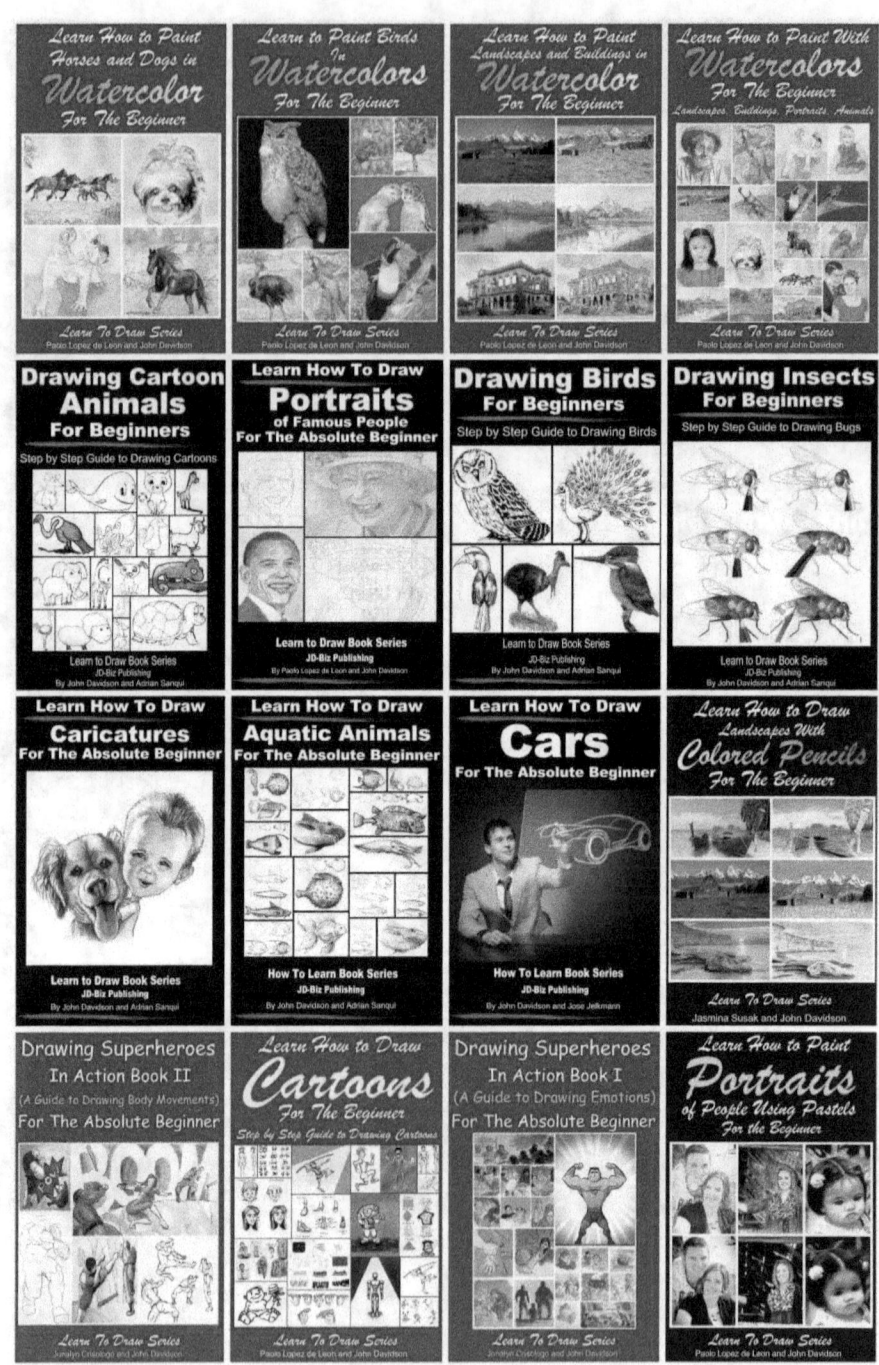

How to Build and Plan Books

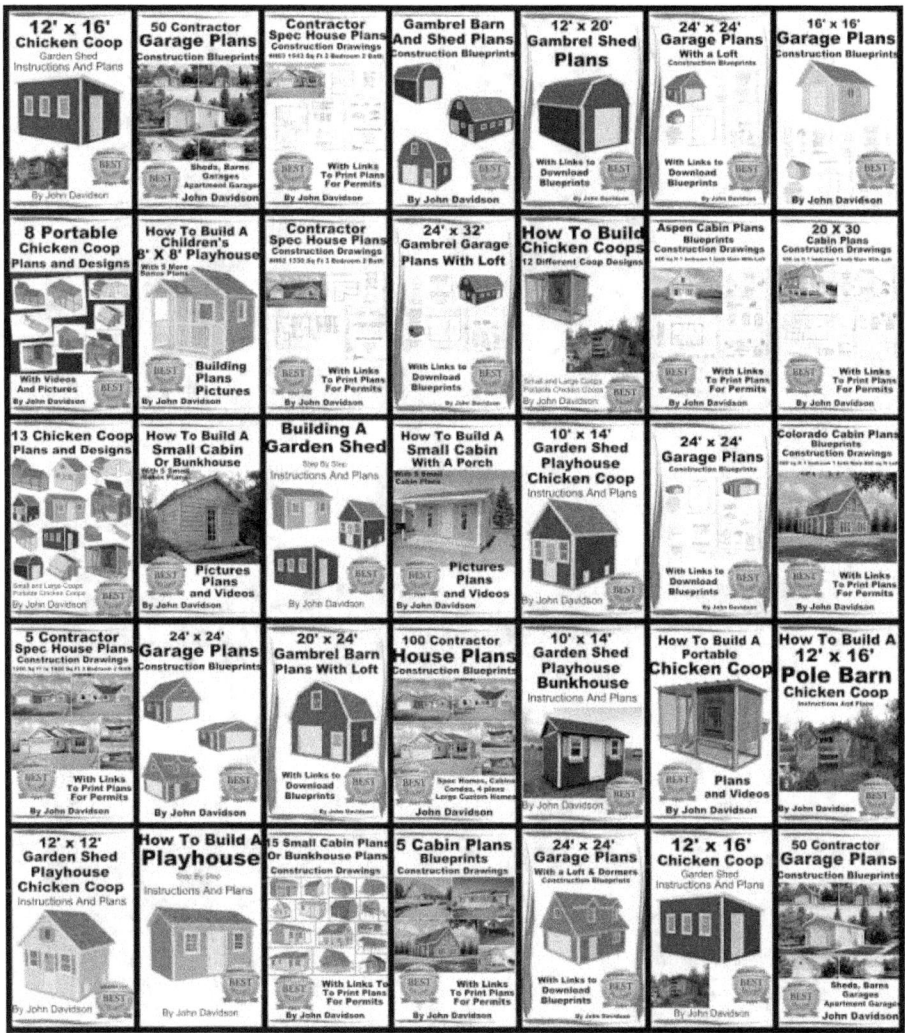

Entrepreneur Book Series

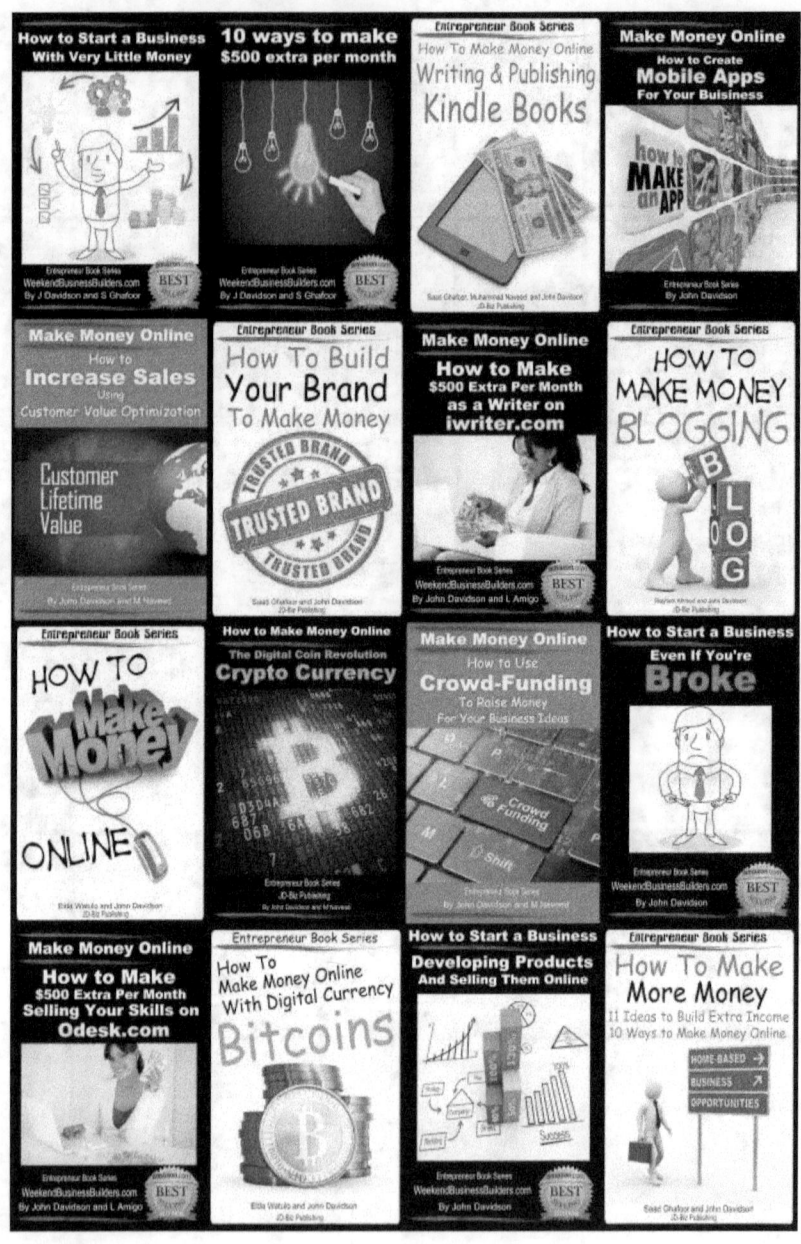

Our books are available at

1. Amazon.com

2. Barnes and Noble

3. Itunes

4. Kobo

5. Smashwords

6. Google Play Books

Download Free Books!

http://MendonCottageBooks.com

Publisher

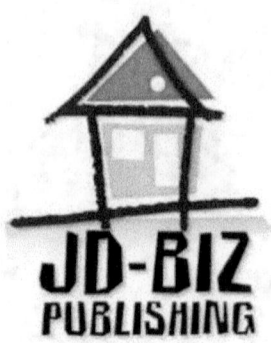

JD-Biz Corp

P O Box 374

Mendon, Utah 84325

http://www.jd-biz.com/

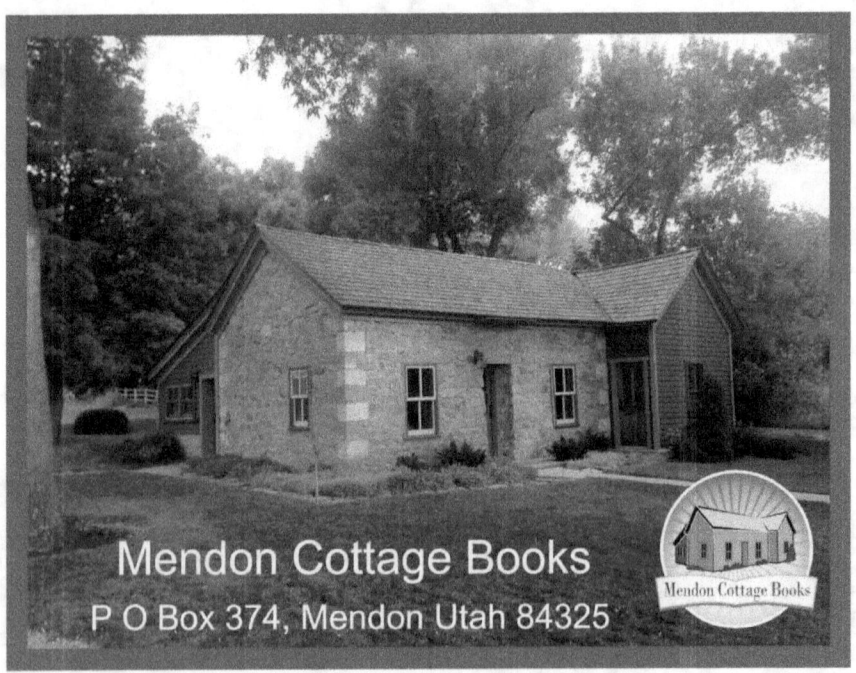

Mendon Cottage Books
P O Box 374, Mendon Utah 84325